The Guide to a Healthy Lifestyle
8 Keys to Unlocking Good Health

I.Nelly Lewis

ISBN-13: 978-1534774346

ISBN-10: 1534774343

Author - I. Nelly Lewis

Help with translation - Orit Davidovich

To my happy family — my dear husband Adam and my two sweet boys: Lee-oz and Eden.

I am so grateful for your unconditional love.

Thank you for supporting me and believing in me every step of the way.

I love you.

Table of Contents

Introduction

Life, what an adventure…

Such a unique opportunity, a fascinating journey.

Rudolf Steiner, the founding father of Anthroposophy, claimed that destiny is an ongoing dialogue between the individual and the world. Individuals can take responsibility for their own destiny and be in dialogue with the world.

Of course, society and divine power (if you believe in one) have always had their share of influence — individuals do not have sole control over their destinies. Nevertheless, as long as we live, we have the choice to take an active part in shaping our own lives: the life we wish for, the life we choose.

Our body is the most precious instrument we have. We all agree health is invaluable, though, in a busy, competitive world, flooded with information and goods, leading a healthy lifestyle is not always easy.

For whatever reason, we do not always find within ourselves enough resolve to resist temptations. We neglect ourselves. We make unhealthy choices instead of those that benefit our physical and emotional present and future health and life.

Unhealthy food, a sedentary lifestyle that neglects the body, high levels of stress, giving in to depression — all those harmful factors, and countless more, confront us.

In fact, almost every single one of us has his or her own persistent stumbling blocks. If only we look closer, we will be able to identify recurring patterns in the way we run into them. One has to say, it is a sad pattern to behold.

Imagine a cartoon character that wakes up each morning only to run into the very same obstacle and then continue to hit against it, time and again. It knows the obstacle is there — it certainly hurts when it runs against it. Perhaps this cartoon character is even angry at itself for doing so. Still, time and again, each time anew, it sets itself up against the same obstacle. Think: a "Tom and Jerry" episode. This could even be funny.

However, where it comes to our own life — our singular opportunity to exist in world full of wonder — funny as it may be, it is nevertheless a sad script. If you are that character that runs against the same obstacle (by means of your own lifestyle choices) and finds it painful, then you are denying yourself the chance to live a full and mindful life.

All those obstacles have their painful consequences, not only in the short but also in the long run.

But then again, what if you simply remove the obstacle? Or bypass it? Choose a different path? Make a different choice? As Jim Rohn once said, truth is simple, for if it were complicated everyone would get it, would they not?

Sometimes it starts from the right call for help. Sometimes you start by building the right framework.

The ego pushes us towards the familiar. Dare I say, You may have even grown "addicted" to that feeling you get after running into the same obstacles. The ego likes familiar places (emotional, sensorial), where change seems impossible and far beyond reach. In many cases, our inability to bring about change invokes a vicious circle of self-deprecation, self-disappointment, self-despair. From that point on, a sense of low self-esteem builds up in the subconscious, which affects self-confidence. This reflects on our daily life, the choices we make, the actions we take, our personal narrative, our relationships, our health, our life, the way we go about things, our level of energy and the way we experience the moment. All this has long-term consequences, of course, whose effect we come to realize only some years later when it is, perhaps, too late. However, now we can still change.

Now is the time. Now is the time to take those steps to improve your life quality. Allow yourself to live with the body you deserve — strong, healthy, in good shape. Let go of your reliance on unhealthy habits, experience tranquillity and maintain a positive mindset. Live life as it should be, the way you would like it to be.

This book is designed to provide you with the tools for recognizing your habits as they are now, to help you come to know the obstacles and patterns you pit yourself against (the ones you wish to change), to provide you with information and tools for accomplishing change.

Do you recognize how important it is to take charge of your own destructive habits? Can you imagine the effect fostering new habits will have? Would you wish to be supported and encouraged to live a healthier, happier life?

I do hope this book speaks to you. I do hope you relate to its ideas and suggestions as they stir you on a path towards a healthier lifestyle.

Lifestyle coaching can be fun.

Even though this is a book, and not an actual lifestyle coaching session, I believe you will find ideas here for a better, healthier, happier life, with a sound and centred body and mind — a life that is the product of a conscious choice.

Change and Changing — Possible!

One of the things I love most in life is the human capacity for learning, which is essentially the ability to change.

I stand in awe of the infinite beauty in learning and the transformation that goes along with it.

What we learn shapes our personality and our life.

When I speak of learning, I speak not only of learning a trade, a musical instrument, a language, or any other skill for that matter. I speak of learning about ourselves, about our own behavioural patterns. Learning is a disciplined practice. Learning happens through trial and error, through practice and repetition. We possess the capacity for learning and instructing ourselves. We possess the capacity for initiating internal change, evolving into a higher self, discovering our life's essence and navigating growth.

Some time ago, a kind woman (82 years of age) arrived at my wellness centre. She brought with her two red tulips — their stems were wrapped at the tip in paper towel and bound in plastic foil — and handed them to me.

We talked for half an hour, more or less. After she had left, I looked at the tulips she had given me. By that point, they seemed already half wilted, limp, their heads drooping, sad.

"That fast?" I wondered. I removed the paper and plastic wrap and set them in a low vase with water. I propped their heavy heads up against the wall and went about my daily business.

Two days later, when I returned to my wellness centre, I found them lying outside the vase in full bloom: erect and proud, as if they were done drinking their fill and decided to leap out the vase for some leisure. I set them back in the vase, this time upright and beautiful, as if a miracle has taken place.

Filled with gratitude, I thought of the woman. I thanked her for the lesson of the tulips she had shared with me.

At times it may seem as if things are not going quite as they should, as if change for the better is not possible, as if all is lost, as if all is over, as if things are as they are and will forever be, as if there is nothing more to do, as if it is best to give in, accept with resignation, ignore, forget, blot out, cast aside, run away.

But, what did the tulips have to say? I believe their message was that by being mindful, by responding to basic needs, with care and compassion, we will carry out one simple truth, we will bring about far-reaching change: what was once withered is now in bloom, what was once dying is now reborn, what has once bowed down is now standing tall.

How beautiful those red tulips are in full bloom. In their full splendour, they fill my heart with hope that each and every one of you may find your way to quench your thirst, to choose those things that give you strength and help you blossom.

Coping with Pain and Disease

Though I am a great believer in our ability to control our lives, assume responsibility for our health choices and, consequently, change the state of our health, I know that, at times, there are greater forces at work. We cannot always do away with or resolve a health issue merely by giving up one particular habit or adopting another.

Despite the great power stored within our minds, we cannot always tap into it in order to do away with or resolve pain or sickness.

Nevertheless, two things can assist us in such circumstances. The first is to accept our condition and set about to address it with proper intervention, for instance, by following the course of treatment prescribed by our physician or by following any other course of action capable of treating our health condition so that it does not get worse and does hopefully get better.

It is not always easy to accept the "gift" that was handed to us without prior warning and beyond our control. Nonetheless, we should not let our health condition put us down and take over our life. Acceptance is the first step to a proper response, one that would allow us to keep on living from a position of strength and competence.

The second thing that can help us directly touches on the first (the first being acceptance). By that I mean our attitude towards our condition and our way of relating to it and to ourselves.

The best way for me to demonstrate this point is with a personal example. I have always had a smooth skin. Short dresses that reveal my legs and arms have always been my outfit of choice. In fact, I have quite the collection of adorable short dresses.

At the age of 37, painful red patches appeared on my elbows that turned out to be a breakout of psoriasis. It is in my genes — my grandmother, mother and uncle all have it. When I told my mother about the dermatologist's diagnosis, she began to cry. I did not understand what made her so emotional. Shortly thereafter, though, I have come to realize these tears were the tears of one who understands what it means to live with a chronic, troubling disease. Soon enough, the breakout on my elbows spread to my legs and other areas of my body and left me feeling helpless and doomed.

The beautiful short dresses were put away. I found myself feeling self-conscious about wearing short outfits that expose affected areas (something of an issue for a Pilates instructor).

Even though I am very much in favour of natural remedies, those natural substances I tried did not make my condition go away, and the more I tried to overlook it, the worse it got. Every time I observed my skin condition, I hated it and felt my life will never be the same. With every visit to a fashion store, I found myself overwhelmed with great sadness, since I felt I was no longer worthy of short dresses, only of those clothes that could hide my psoriatic body.

The disease requires care daily, which includes applying special creams and ointments. It demands special attention, time and effort on my part. So long as I resisted it, sought to overlook it, hated it, neglected its treatment, my condition got worse. It certainly affects mood and quality of life, when your body is itching and painful.

Once I accepted I have this "gift", I started taking care of it regularly. Now, my toddler son loves to apply the cream over my skin while playing "doctor". The more I reminded myself to take care of it and not feel so bad about it (with the help of NLP, as well), my condition got better.

I decided I do not wish for the disease to stop me from adding to my collection of short dresses or determine my choices and sought creative solutions (such as stockings). I started working on coping with the sense of shame the disease had brought about, so that I may overcome it.

The disease will forever be inside me. At present, it has no cure. However, I decided to see it in a different light — as a gift, a gift that reminds me, first and foremost, to be thankful, every moment, for each thing that functions properly in my body, a gift that allows me to come to terms with imperfections within me, with defects, and find within me the compassion and self-love to take care of myself without hate, judgement or sadness.

I do not let it have undue power over me. At present, I regard it much the same as wearing contact lenses. It presents me with the opportunity to give myself time for self-maintenance and to develop my self-confidence. It encourages me to reflect on issues of body image and social standards, to deal with imperfection and to welcome sincerity into my life.

There is a beautiful folk tale about the flower with the golden heart. It tells the story of a young boy's journey in search of a cure for his sick mother. The doctors have already despaired. Only one old doctor says the only way to save the boy's mother would be with the help of the flower with the golden heart: once she smells it, she would be cured. However, this precious flower grows somewhere far away and so the boy must go on a true adventure. In the end he finds the flower and brings it back to his mother, she smells it and regains perfect health.

I love this story and believe there is a flower with a golden heart to heal my skin, perhaps in the form of a mushroom. I am planning at some point to go on a journey to find a real cure for my skin issues. I see these issues as a call for a quest, a journey, an adventure — and so it is.

I do not know what health issues you deal with — perhaps temporary, perhaps chronic. Whatever the case may be, I invite you to search for ways to take care of yourself better, more compassionately. It is your body's call for love and care. It is the opportunity to discover your strength, to overcome the negative and grab hold of the good.

When we experience pain, it is a great challenge. Therefore, I invite you to allow yourself to seek and get help, should you need it.

Be Mindful of Diagnoses and Prognoses

I am not a physician, and I do not presume to be a source of medical authority. However, as one who is passionate about health, who has been studying health and wellbeing for over 25 years, I place great emphasis on medical consultation — in matters of health, I always refer my coachees to seek advice from the medical establishment. There is no doubt, medicine helps us tremendously — it is crucial.

However, I have run into many cases of false diagnosis, or cases in which doctors' opinions turned out to be wrong. Since doctors are a source of authority, there is a tendency to accept their words as definite, when they express their opinion or provide diagnosis (the line between the two is not always clear, something we should be mindful of).

Here, I call upon you to exercise discretion, to seek a second opinion (or a third, or a fourth) and trust your intuition. In the end of the day, what we accept as truth, and believe it to be so, will determine the course of our life. Where a false diagnosis is concerned, it can truly rob you of your potential and ability to live your life, healthy and positive.

Often times, people come to me for a Pilates session claiming they suffer from chronic neck or back pain. "Chronic" is defined to be an ongoing condition that never goes away. When you accept "chronic" as a qualifier for you condition, you reinforce and reaffirm its chronic status and, in this way, deprive yourself of the possibility to resolve, improve

or heal it.

There are many examples out there for misdiagnoses and wrong opinions. I will never forget that time when a gynaecologist told me I had polycystic ovary syndrome — I was only 15 or 16, at the time. What a scary term for a young woman to hear from a gynaecologist she has just seen for the first time. When I asked my gynaecologist what implications such diagnosis entails, the doctor replied I would run into difficulty trying to conceive and would, most likely, require medication to help me get pregnant.

The gynaecologist was a well-known, renowned expert. I came out of that appointment shattered. I remember myself crying, struck by the prognosis the doctor had imparted.

Years later, when I decided to have children, I refused to accept the gynaecologist's "prognosis". I encouraged myself to have faith in my own fertility and the body's natural function. I was pregnant with both my first and second child a few months after making the decision, without any further intervention. I believe, had I made the choice to stand by the doctor's prognosis, it would have had its impact, and I certainly would not have become a mother that easily.

Dr Richard Bandler (co-developer of NLP) was told he would not be able to walk again and would spend the rest of his life bound to a wheelchair. He refused to accept the prognosis and rehabilitated himself with the power of faith and thought. Today he walks as normal as ever.

There are countless such examples.

What Is Our Health Made Of?

What Is the Problem?

What is our health made of? What makes us healthy and full of vitality? You probably agree with me that health is imminent. Nevertheless, it is not always easy to answer these questions. It is harder still to nurture our health regularly, day in, day out.

Here are 8 key factors to good health:

1. Staying hydrated

2. Stress management

3. Physical activity

4. Weight management

5. Social connections

6. Meditation and prayer

7. Overcoming unhealthy habits

8. Leisure / Creativity / Personal Development

Do you lead a healthy lifestyle? Would you like to get a clearer picture of where you stand in terms of your health?

Let me present to you the health chart exercise. Consider the health chart below. Score each key factor in the chart from "1" to "10" according to your level of satisfaction with this aspect in your life. The number "1" designates the lowest level of satisfaction and the number "10" designates the highest level (located on the outer ring of the wheel). Once you are done with your scores, connect all the dots (there should be 8 of them) with a curved line, to create your own inner circle capturing how you are doing on the whole.

Your Health Chart

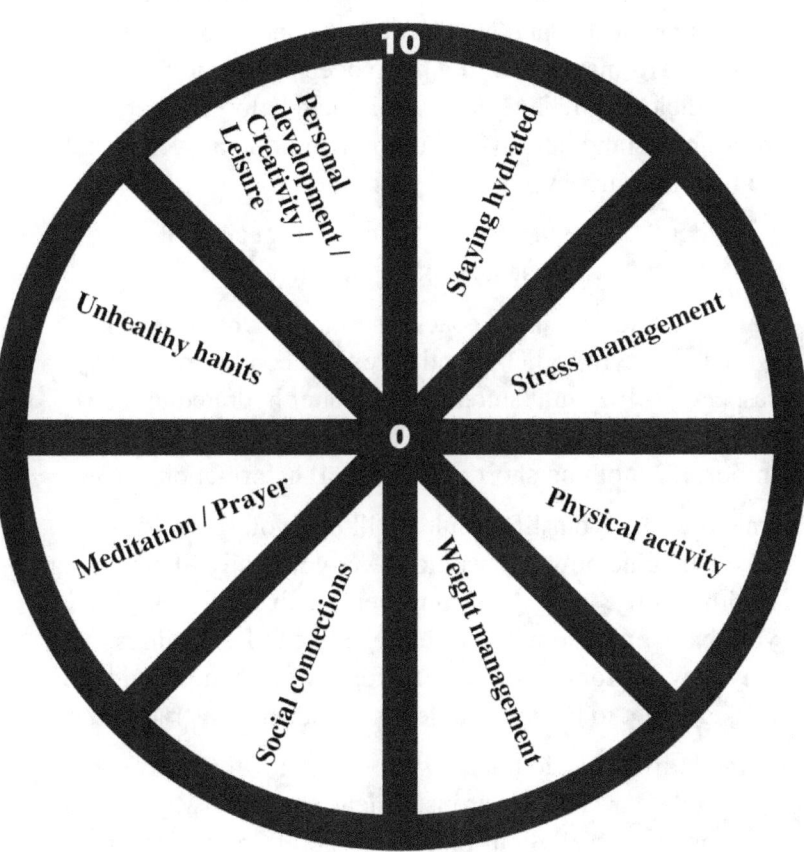

Now consider, if this were a wheel, would it be rolling? Does it appear round? Of course, if we were now in a coaching session, we would be discussing each key factor, in order to examine it closely and gain a deeper understanding. Naturally, in a book format, our ability to go deeper is limited. Nevertheless, I believe this exercise can help you sharpen your understanding of your current condition as well as help you clarify where you would wish it to be.

Consider the 8 key factors in the chart, especially those where you scored low. What steps can you take to optimise them?

I am proud to say, those coachees of mine who first arrive with a "flat tyre" quickly optimize their condition in many respects — they quit smoking, get better hydrated, get on a healthy diet, make new friends and more — the change is not minor; it is nothing short of genuine transformation.

Imagine what your life would be like, if you scored "10" in each. Imagine how that would affect your daily life and your health and life in the long run, even the lives of those dear to you. Now imagine what it would be like to keep things the way they are for one more year, for two, for ten. Would you consider that to be unbearable? Is it not truly destructive?

Some individuals do not do well, since they themselves do not feel well. Our body is our instrument, the same way that our brain is the vessel of our thoughts. Therefore, treat your body as a temple — not a tent, not a hut, not a sleeping bag — a temple!

In the following few pages I will briefly share with you some information regarding each key factor in the health chart. Surely, each person is different. Each individual has his or her own needs and a different way of going about reaching the optimum. This book is certainly not a substitute for a training process. Nonetheless, I find it useful to share information concerning the various key factors in the chart: to clarify why each is important and how each can be improved upon. I invite you to read it all or choose those sections that are relevant to you.

Staying Hydrated

How much water do you drink a day? Too much? Too little? Just the right amount? Water plays a significant role in our level of vitality. Water constitutes a crucial ingredient to a healthy lifestyle. In this chapter, I will provide a number of "dry" facts about water and staying hydrated.

Why do we need water?

As Leonardo da Vinci said, "Water is the driving force of all nature". Our body cannot function without water, the same way a car cannot run without petrol. In fact, each element of human anatomy and physiology depends on water for proper function.

In addition to preventing dehydration, water contributes to our mood: our body feels good and our sense of energy increases. Not only does it sustain life, water has many health benefits in nourishing the skin. Like any other organ, the skin is negatively impacted by dehydration. With sufficient hydration, the skin heals and appears younger. Water promotes skin moisture and boosts skin elasticity as well as rejuvenates skin cells and tissues.

Moreover, it is vital for detoxing, strengthening the immune system and reducing health risks. Research establishes that drinking enough water reduces the risk of cancer, asthma, and hypertension as well as supports weight loss by supressing appetite.

How do we lose water?

The body loses water through urine, respiration and sweat. We lose more water when active than while sitting. Diuretic drugs, caffeine and alcohol may enhance body water loss. Therefore, loss of fluids must be offset with fluid intake from food or drink.

What are the sign of mild dehydration?

The symptoms of mild dehydration include: thirst, pain to muscles and joints, lower back pain, headache and constipation.

Is it possible to drink too much?

As a matter of fact, yes. Excessive fluid intake may lead to water poisoning — the result of taking in a large amount of fluids with low Nitrogen content (as with mineral water). An individual with normal kidney function on a low-nitrate diet will suffer severe water poisoning if he or she drinks more than 1.8 litres of water in one go, while an individual not on a low-nitrate diet will experience the same consequences when he or she exceeds 3 litres.

How much water is enough?

What constitutes sufficient water intake changes according to climate (hot or temperate), level of physical activity and a person's health. Personally, I make sure to drink 2 litres of fluids a day. There is no definite scientific indication that drinking 8 cups of fluids per day is the right amount. Nonetheless, I recommend you regard it as a guideline.

If it is that simple, why is everyone not following this advice?

Insufficient fluid intake triggers a mechanism in the brain that translates into a sense of thirst. Not everyone pays that signal due attention. Our lives are rife with distractions. Unless you make it a habit, it is easy to "forget" to drink sufficiently. Moreover, many soft drinks today contain plenty of caffeine and sugar. Though they are categorized as fluids, they do not contribute much as far as nutritional value or hydration are concerned. Some individuals do not appreciate the taste of water and find it hard to drink it in its pure form.

What can be done about it?

Naturally, this is a personal matter, depending on your schedule, diet, and lifestyle. To answer the question generally, I would recommend you examine your fluid intake habits. Could you reduce your caffeine or alcohol intake? Could you add a little more water to your glass each time you drink — just a little more or just one more glass? Could you set aside time for fluid intake? I always drink water first thing in the morning.

If you do not appreciate the taste of water or wish to spruce it up a little, I recommend infusing it with fruit for a few minutes to give it that fresh, fun zest. Cucumber-flavoured water is truly refreshing and so is lemon-flavoured water. If you wish to go for something sweeter, try using apples or peaches. You are welcome to experiment with all sorts of fruit, check what works best for you. Nevertheless, I would avoid sweetened bottled water.

Before we move on, how about you take a break to sip a glass of water?

Stress Management

How is it that we can always find new reasons to get stressed? Stress comes easily and intensifies easily. Stress increases the level of the hormone Cortisol. Research indicates that high levels of Cortisol, sustained over time as a result of prolonged stress, exhaust the body and damage health in the long run. Stress accelerates aging and increases appetite. It causes insomnia, skin problems, osteoporosis and more.

Almost anything may cause stress. It results from various factors that change from one individual to the next. For some individuals, in some cases, merely thinking about a certain issue, or a number of minor yet exacerbating issues that accumulate over time, may result in stress.

Some of the most common causes for stress are: family issues, financial strife, disease, work, premenstrual syndrome, too little time for completing assignments, sense of boredom, moving houses, relationships or divorce, events such as unexpected pregnancy or death in the family, inconsiderate neighbours, uncertainty (for instance, when expecting lab, exam or interview results) and many more.

It may also be the case that an individual would experience stress, frustration, anxiety or depression with no apparent causes in evidence.

The Impact of Stress on Our Daily Behaviour

Some consequences of stress interfere with body function, complicate thoughts and feelings and disrupt behaviour. A study published in 2012 pointed to the fact that parents who induce stress in their children increase their child's likelihood of suffering from overweight, learning disabilities or behavioural issues.

Conditions that invoke stress in humans include factors that contribute not only to stress but also to poor physical health. Stress may be expressed in any one of the following symptoms: muscle pain or spasms, nervous ticks, loss of sexual appetite, headaches, biting nails, fainting fits, lack of sleep, hypertension, sensitive stomach, weak immune system or a needle pricking sensation. Stress may result in heart diseases or ulcers.

Normally, in stressful circumstances, individuals experience one of two primal impulses: either "fight" or "flight". This is the nervous system's way of responding to a threatening event. The body produces larger quantities of Adrenalin, which stimulates the heart, tenses up the muscles, activates sweat glands and produces alertness. All these assist in helping the individual protect his or herself from harm or challenge.

However, where it comes to excessive prolonged stress, it is best to do without it.

Treating Stress

You can choose to tackle stress using one or more of the following approaches: self-help (altering cognitions), professional help (health coaching, alternative therapies) and medication.

Medication can certainly contribute to relaxation. I must admit, one time, when I lived in a conflict zone at a time of war I took Oxazepam to help myself calm down. In the end, I chose a natural means for eliminating that type of stress — getting out of that danger zone. However, there is a risk involved in taking medication. It could be that its sole contribution turns out to be concealing stress instead of helping the individual cope over the long run.

Where "mild" stress is concerned — the type of stress that results from intrusive thoughts or needless worry — there are alternative ways for controlling stress level: meditation, relaxation, reassessment of your situation, social support, better time management and more.

Throughout my career as a lifestyle coach, I helped many coachees to reduce their levels of stress and experience more comfortable, peaceful lives in various ways. Some coachees found NLP and guided imagery to be helpful in disengaging from stressful situations, observing them from the outside, viewing them from a different, calmer perspective with a greater degree of control. Many made the choice to adopt habits that promote stress release, such as meditation or exercise.

If stress is an issue you deal with, perhaps it may seem impossible to get it under control. Certainly, when you are anxious and alone it is not always easy to sit back for a moment and listen to your breathing, from inhale to exhale. Whatever the case may be, I can assure you, the road to relaxation begins once you find a method that works well for you, a technique you can perform easily. So long as it is helpful, it is the starting point for major improvement.

Exercise

Now it is time to relax. We move to physical exercise and nutrition (two of my favourite key factors). Both contribute remarkably to quality of life. When done properly, each quickly invokes a wonderful emotional and physical sensation.

Why physical exercise?

Physical exercise benefits many aspects of health: reduces the risk of heart disease, stroke or diabetes, prevents certain types of cancer, builds up bone mass, strengthens muscles, raises energy levels, develops lung capacity and diminishes the risk for accidents and fractures. Exercise burns calories and supports weight loss. It boosts body image and self-image.

Notably, it facilitates the reduction of stress, tension and depression, elevates mood by releasing Endorphins (hormones that have an effect similar to Opiates, resulting in a pleasant sense of "high") and helps with falling asleep and general quality of sleep.

Many studies conducted during the last few years demonstrate that exercise improves brain function, especially as it relates to tasks that require concentration, coordination and memory.

Yet another advantage of exercise is found in emotional resilience and self-confidence. Each time you tap into your inner resources overcoming an obstacle, you connect to your centre, that immense reservoir of strength that is within you.

There are two types of physical exercise: aerobic and anaerobic.

What is aerobic exercise?

Running, swimming, cycling, spinning, skiing, aerobics and zumba classes: these are all aerobic activities. By definition, an aerobic activity is an activity sustained over an extended period of time that involves the concentrated effort of all muscle groups. During such activity, oxygen consumption intensifies and heart rate increases, which facilitates heightened fat metabolism. The recommended level of aerobic physical activity is twice a week (and, for those who wish to lose weight, three to five times a week).

What are the benefits of aerobic exercise?

Aerobic exercise is considered the number one activity recommended for disease prevention. It reduces the risk of cardiac and vascular diseases. Such activity strengthens the cardiac muscle and balances blood sugar levels. It lowers the risk of cancer and boosts function for all physiological systems. Aerobic exercise develops cardiovascular endurance and allows us to stay fit.

What is anaerobic exercise?

Anaerobic exercise is a short-duration, high-intensity activity that utilizes energy stored in the muscles. Its name refers to the fact that oxygen consumption is not involved in the process — hence the term "an-aerobic". Activities such as yoga, Pilates (my favourite activity), weightlifting and floor workout are considered anaerobic.

What are the benefits of anaerobic exercise?

Anaerobic exercise develops muscle and body strength. Such activity turns sugar into the source of energy necessary for building up muscle mass at the expense of fat mass. Anaerobic exercise is needed for toning muscles during weight loss. It is recommended that aerobic and anaerobic exercise be combined together. When exercised in synergy, you truly promote general good health. Combining both exercise regimes can vastly improve body tone and appearance.

I recommend starting with aerobic exercise and then moving onto anaerobic exercise, for example, starting with a vigorous brisk walk and following with Pilates (I especially enjoy MOTR Pilates, a combination of both anaerobic and aerobic exercise).

Before you start, it is first important that you visit your doctor for a general check-up, especially if you have been experiencing pain. It is vital that you follow up on it before you begin exercising. In many cases, exercise can put an end to pain such as back, shoulder, knee or neck pain as well as alleviate muscle tension and headaches. It goes without saying, exercise should not be pursued if you experience pain throughout. Continuing to do so may only make things worse; it would make it more likely for you experience pain in the future.

Still, there is a difference between "good pain" and "bad pain". Good pain is a sign that you are working to get yourself stronger, while bad pain is your body asking you to stop whatever movement you are doing — that movement is not making things better.

In our day and age, there are many programs and videos available online. Still, I, personally, recommend taking part in an actual class led by a professional instructor who would make sure you are doing the exercises correctly. Once you are confident in your ability to perform exercises safely and correctly, you may take advantage of the wonders of technology for this purpose. However, please exercise both body and caution when going online for random exercise routines.

Unfortunately, some videos offer false information with exercises that may do more harm

than good.

How many times a week?

Many studies indicate that the individuals who benefit most from exercise are those who perform it daily. Regrettably, many find it hard to dedicate that much time for such an extensive exercise regime. The recommendation is, therefore, to exercise at least four times a week. Beginners should aim for three, with one day of rest, at least, in between two consecutive training sessions. A fourth session may be added after a few months of regular training.

The most important thing is to start — to start with some form of exercise, be it aerobic or anaerobic. A single Pilates class a week, a single swimming lesson, walking to work instead of driving, using the stairs instead of the lift: so long as you choose an activity that seems fun and exciting but also fits your physical needs. It is recommended that you fix a designated time for training on your calendar, the same day and hour. This would make it easier for you to integrate exercise into your busy schedule.

General advice

Do not exercise immediately after a meal. In contrast, make sure not to exercise having had nothing to eat for an extended period of time. Depending on the type of activity, it is generally recommended that you eat no later than an hour and a half before your training session begins. Drink water in abundance before and after.

Are You Familiar With Pilates?

In case you are not familiar with Pilates, allow me to introduce to you this outstanding exercise method together with my enthusiastic recommendation that you try it out for yourself to see what it can do for you. Millions of people around the world have fallen in love with Pilates — a healthy addiction that has transformed lives and keeps advancing physical and mental health. I am speaking here from personal experience.

This method was formerly known as "Contrology". The term was designed to evoke its primary purpose: to give the trainee firm control over his or her body. Eventually, the name that did take hold was "Pilates" after its founder Joseph Pilates, an athlete and rehabilitation genius who established and developed the method.

Pilates comprises a scheme of exercises and movements that combine muscle workout together with flexibility, coordination and aerobics. The method releases tension away from overloaded joints and increases blood flow and oxygen supply throughout the body. This synthesis between enhanced blood flow together with a stronger body, a wider range of motion and an improved muscular balance leads to a healthy body that moves with grace and ease. Pilates strengthens, flexes and releases the body away from an unhealthy posture. It helps its trainees to heal from back and neck pain as well as various joint problems. It eases and releases tension and fatigue.

Doctors, physiotherapists, dancers and athletes appreciate Pilates both for its healing power and as an intelligent physical exercise scheme that supports good body maintenance. The method is popular worldwide. Its broad range of exercises, along with the equipment that supports it, generates countless many training options. Therefore, it is never lacking in variety and always challenging.

Here is a testimonial by one of my clients, Vicky L.:

> "Pilates can be transformative. […] I have been learning how to move and to listen to my body in a new way.
>
> When I started Pilates, I was struggling to control various symptoms, including severe back and limb pain and a type of chronic inflammation in my pelvic floor. I'm very fortunate in having the opportunity to work with Nelly Lewis. Pilates is a powerful tool; for that very reason, it has to be taught well. Perhaps especially if you're struggling with your health, you need someone to be aware of that and to adapt the postures and movements to your particular needs. In my case, Nelly's deeply sensitive approach to Pilates – as both a technique and a *relation* to one's own body – has had an enormous impact. Much of my limb and back pain has disappeared; the pelvic pain is improving, I even lost weight without a change in my diet.
>
> For me, Pilates has inspired nothing less than a new relation to my body. Not only in terms of my health (though that, of course, is crucial). But Pilates has also changed my sense of being in the world."

If you are currently suffering from pain and would like to learn how you can get rid of it, even before starting with Pilates, join me for my webinar "How to Reduce Aches and Pains Even Before Starting to Practice Pilates". To find it online, go to   www.nellylewis.com/webinars

Weight Management

The term "weight management" involves both attaining and preserving body weight within a range that promotes health. Weight management concerns itself not only with weight *per se* but also with body fat percentage.

The key to adopting a healthy lifestyle, losing weight or maintaining your desired body weight is in changing eating habits and opting for a better relationship with food and yourself. More often than not, food craving (the unhealthy kind) is triggered at times of emotional imbalance (as a result of stress, boredom, loneliness etc.). During such times, food acts both as a comforter and as an occasion for negative self-talk.

This type of eating is known as "emotional eating" and it can jeopardise your efforts to lose weight. It tends to involve excessive eating of unhealthy food rich in calories, such as sweets, snacks, processed food or high-fat foods.

Emotional eating is eating as a means to supress or to soothe negative emotions, such as stress, anger, fear, boredom, sadness or loneliness. Day-to-day life problems can trigger negative emotions that result in adopting emotional eating as a habit, which can interfere with your efforts to lose weight or negatively affect your vitality, health and general mood. Such problems may include work-related stress, fatigue, financial stress, conflicted relationships, health problems and more.

In fact, your emotions may have become inextricably linked to your eating habits, so much so that they automatically dictate your eating patterns. Eating also serves as a distraction. If you are worried over a future eventuality, for instance, you may settle for eating comfort food instead of dealing with the source of stress.

I invite you to pay attention to those circumstances in which you use emotional eating. What can you say about these circumstances? When do they occur? Why do they occur? What types of food are involved? It would be interesting to know why you choose certain types of food as comforting. Do you happen to remember the first time you ate these? Often times, your particular choices have to do with childhood experiences, where certain types of food were experienced as comforting or made you feel loved.

Feelings that make you overindulge — eat not in response to physical hunger but in response to emotional hunger — give rise to new unpleasant feelings that get you to overindulge again. It is a vicious cycle.

The good news is that, if you are one of those who struggle with emotional eating, you can take steps to re-establish control over your eating habits to facilitate healthier ones that go hand in hand with your wish to live a healthy, positive life.

Why eating habits and not diet?

As studies demonstrate, only a change in eating habits can sustain weight loss over the long term. My view on the matter is that short-term fad diets are not only unhealthy but also leave little room for the type of understanding and development needed to bring about real change that could be sustained over time.

A diet usually determines what you may or may not eat. When trying to avoid a certain type of food, it is more likely that you will end up craving exactly that food which you are not allowed to eat. The minute your diet comes to a close, you are likely to reach for "forbidden" food. Until that moment arrives, you will likely stress and torment yourself — the victim of your diet goals.

I favour the one-step-at-a-time approach. This way you may move forward, confident, independent and aware, while recognizing your limitations and needs, so that your choices are in harmony with your lifestyle and schedule without restrictions or prohibitions.

My approach:

1. Awareness

First things first: knowing what is healthy and what is not. Nowadays, there is considerable public awareness for health. On the other hand, many foods marketed as healthy, found in supermarket aisles, are, in fact, far from being so (consider, for example, power bars, fruits and vegetables sprayed with chemicals and more).

It is worth your while to learn more about nutrition to help you decide on your food combinations. For example, Iron is found in green vegetables in significant quantities. For your body to better absorb Iron, vitamin C is needed. The latter can be found in tomatoes, red sweet peppers, cantaloupes and kiwis. In contrast, combining Iron with dairy products significantly reduces its absorption.

This is a fascinating topic, worthy of an entire volume. In this book, however, I only intend to give you a little taste of it. If you believe you are not acquainted enough with healthy food and cooking, the easiest thing to do would be to visit a bookstore nearby and find a book on healthy cooking to get yourself started. I am certain, you will soon find out which healthy foods may substitute unhealthy ones in your daily diet. Healthy foods will help you nurture your body and mind with beneficial energy and maintain a healthy body weight.

2. Supportive environment

Establish a supportive environment for yourself. Make sure your kitchen is stocked up with healthy food, so that when you open the fridge, you will find a healthy fresh fruit dessert or some other healthy snack (for example, dates rolled in sesame seeds) instead of cake bought at the supermarket rich in vegetable oil. If you feel like snacking, make sure to have popcorn available (the kind you yourself make from dried kernels) instead of a bag of chips, perhaps even try satiating the urge with seasonal greens (preferably organic). You can make your own ice cream instead of buying one at the store. Examples are plenty!

3. Eat mindfully

Mindful eating makes food taste better. It allows you to turn into a gourmet food critic. You enjoy each minute you eat mindfully, while being aware of your body, paying special attention to when eating for nourishment ends and emotional eating begins.

Eating mindfully has a great power in allowing you to make a real change where it comes to nutrition and better weight management. Mindful eating is one of the best well-tested ways to lose weight. It works without having to put up a struggle — without a diet — to get rid of automatic eating and gain control over unhealthy over-eating.

There are many ways for you to train yourself to eat mindfully. You can start practicing it with something small, a piece of fruit, perhaps. Here are a few possible stages to mindful eating.

Say "grace".

A wise person once said: when you eat, just eat. Be sure to dedicate time solely for eating. Avoid eating while watching television or doing any other activity (talking on the phone, scrolling through social media). Before you start eating, take a short pause to examine your food: observe its colours, shapes and textures, savour its scents, think of the journey its ingredients made only to reach your plate. You may say a prayer if you wish.

Eat whatever you feel like.

When working with clients on obtaining a healthy weight, I always tell them to eat whatever their heart desires. Do not deny yourself any type of food. Otherwise, you might end up craving it. Soon enough, you might find yourself gobbling up not only too much but also your own feelings of guilt.

Eat when you are hungry.

Learn to identify when you are experiencing hunger as a physical sensation rather than an emotional one, meaning, hunger resulting from an emotional need. Be sure to eat when you are hungry, not when you are, in fact, not hungry, neither when you are starving.

Stop eating when you are full.

When you eat mindfully you know to stop when you are full (even when there is plenty left on the plate). Eating mindfully frees you from gobbling down food uncontrollably.

Eat slowly.

Studies show it takes about 20 minutes from the moment food is consumed till its digested by-products reach the blood stream to produce a sense of satiation. When you eat too quickly you end up swallowing more than you actually need so that feeling satiated arrives too late. Eating slowly contributes both to mindful eating and to a well-timed sense of satiation.

Chew your food seeking to kindle the senses. Sometimes, I recommend clients use chopsticks, especially when they are not accustomed to (when they are, I recommend holding them in the non-dominant hand or, alternately, laying down the cutlery between each bite).

4. Beliefs and cognitions

Pay attention to your inner dialogue. Is it positive? Do your thoughts support your weight management mission? Do you tell yourself, when you look in the mirror, how overweight you look? Do you tell yourself, each time you eat, that nothing will ever work, that you are doomed to stay overweight? Such thoughts undermine your success, since they may lead you to despair and give in, and consequently go for unhealthy, unmindful eating.

Here is a quote by James Allen:

> "A man is literally what he thinks, his character being the complete sum of all his thoughts."

Nowadays, there is growing awareness to the importance of positive thinking in framing a clear, positive picture of your goals and maintaining that positive picture.

Here is one example of a short exercise that can help you frame a positive picture and maintain a positive image of weight management. Imagine what it would be like once you have accomplished your weight goals. What are you wearing? How are you moving about? Fill your brain with encouraging thoughts: "I am becoming thinner moment by moment", "I choose to eat mindfully", "I look great". You may post encouraging phrases at different locations around your house, little sticky notes to remind you to think positively or compliments to encourage you to move forward with ease and confidence on the path to achieving your goals.

On this issue, I assist coachees with NLP and guided imagery. I usually prepare a personalized recording for the coachee based on our mutual sessions and designed specifically to match the coachee's needs. The coachee may listen to it whenever he or she feels the need, whenever he or she finds it helpful. The path to weight management can be enjoyable and satisfying, at the end of which you will achieve your desired weight and the body you are proud of.

The time needed for losing weight changes from one individual to the other. Each process is unique. Each individual has his or her own path, his or her own metabolism. The fundamental principles remain the same, though: mindful eating, positive thinking and exercise are the three key components that ensure success.

In this chapter I mainly focused on overweight. However, lifestyle coaching is also designed for the opposite condition: underweight, anorexia or any other body image issue.

Meditation or Prayer

Whether you believe in a higher power or not, whether you choose to pray or meditate, both meditation and prayer help you create a peaceful time for getting in touch with your genuine self, listening to your inner wishes.

The effects of meditation and prayer are invaluable to our quality of life. They facilitate stress reduction, increase positivity, allow us to appreciate what we have, rejuvenate energy and afford us better control over our responses, our emotional state and our sense of presence.

When you meditate, you clear your head of pestering thoughts about your job or other day-to-day affairs. Your head becomes a clean slate. All becomes clean and peaceful. It is the time to stop and examine things from the outside using a fresh perspective.

A person may spend an entire life searching for happiness and not see it is right under his or her nose, just as it is, requiring no interference. It is so easy to feel as if something is missing, to focus on what is lacking. Meditation encourages us to clear room in our heads, to stop thinking and start connecting with what we do have — with our life.

As with anything else, meditation requires practice. The more you practice meditation the further you reinforce the positive effects listed above, so much so that, at some point, you will find yourself able to meditate as you go about your daily routine: while you are working, while you are spending time with your children, while you are having a conversation.

A Harvard University study clearly indicated that those who practice meditation not only feel better but also see an actual transformation to brain structure. Their positive, calm feelings linger over time.

Nevertheless, you might not find it easy to practice meditation, whether because you feel you have too little time or adequate space for the purpose, or because you have once had an experience with meditation that made you think it was not right for you. Perhaps you are ready to try out meditation and wish to deepen your understanding of it or do more of it.

Whatever the case may be, I recommend starting with a short session, just a few minutes long. It is important the form of meditation you choose be easy and comfortable for you. You could then increase its duration, little by little, if you feel the need to do so.

Find the meditation technique that fits you best: while sitting, in motion or through prayer. There are so many types of techniques. Surely, you will find one that suits you.

I would say, meditation is precious time well spent.

It is astonishing, how the search for a state of emptiness, the search for a void, can recharge us with so much energy, wisdom, positivity and power.

When you consider your life calmly, when you clear your head of thoughts (a brain cleansing, so to speak), you make room for something new — a fresh, calm and peaceful observation. Meditation helps you reconnect with yourself and listen to your subconscious. It promotes better, more positive thinking and better decision-making. In short, meditation improves your life quality.

If you wish to get inspired to meditate, I recommend reading "Super Rich" by Russel Simmons. In case I were already able to inspire you to meditate at this very moment, I recommend the website http://www.omvana.com, where you will find a wealth of meditation techniques designed for various levels of style and experience.

Enjoy your meditation.

Overcoming Unhealthy Habits

Do you have unhealthy habits — habits you know or feel are harmful, habits that pose a risk to your health and life quality — but hold on to them regardless?

The most common, widespread unhealthy habits are smoking, alcohol drinking, using drugs and unhealthy eating.

Perhaps you have some other unhealthy habit you wish to change, such as drinking coffee, biting your nails, a tendency to lose your temper quickly, a destructive relationship or any other such habit.

All unhealthy habits are the result of some pattern of thought. They can be changed. The only necessary condition for instigating change is a genuine wish to put an end to that particular behavioural pattern and a willingness to cope with momentary discomfort while achieving that goal.

Many hold fast to some justification for not making the change (also known as an excuse). For example, some claim they are physically addicted (to Nicotine, to alcohol). From my own personal experience and from working with clients, change is far simpler than what it appears to be. The power of mind over body is far greater than we think.

Without going into too much detail, I can attest to the fact that putting an end to unhealthy habits is doable, for example where it comes to smoking. Clients I work with usually stop smoking within four sessions. I myself used to be a heavy smoker (to the point that the cigarette became my sixth finger). At the age of 23, I managed to quit smoking after reading the book "The Emotions of daily life and their maintenance" by Ph.D. Ilan Shalif and friends.

In my work with clients, I combine lessons learned from my own personal experience together with NLP techniques, while tailoring my sessions to fit the client's needs.

Perhaps you have already come to the conclusion that the different key factors in your health chart affect one another. It stands to reason that a person who enjoys a good social life, a healthy diet, sufficient hydration, regular exercise and meditation is less likely to find refuge from reality in alcohol or drug consumption.

In the process towards optimized health, we move forward simultaneously on several fronts. As it improves, each key factor in your health chart facilitates the improvement of other factors, making such improvement less demanding even.

Social Connections

In today's world of social media, some individuals find themselves spending more time in front of the screen than in front of other human beings. Those social connections that come about or are supported through media cannot replace true friendships. A true human connection is a form of mutual support and assistance at times of need.

According to psychiatrist Robert Waldinger, the fourth consecutive director of a fascinating Harvard study that has been following 724 people for over 75 years throughout the entire span of their life, from their teenage years to old age, quality relationships keep us healthy and happy. The main points featured in his TED talk are:

1. Good social connections are good for us, while loneliness is fatal. Individuals who stay connected to family, friends and the community at large are healthier. Not only that, they also live longer. In contrast, individuals who remain alone and isolated (who feel they do not have enough social connections) are less happy, their health declines, the state of their brain deteriorates and they end up living a shorter life.

2. Quality of social connections is important. It is not enough to have a connection just for the sake of having one. Social connections should be real, good and sincere. The study demonstrates that those individuals who were the most satisfied with their relationships at 50 were also the healthiest at 80.

3. Good connections of the type we feel we could fall back on at hard times, protect not only our body but also our brain, for example, memory remains sharper and clearer.

Social connections are a crucial ingredient to health and wellbeing. There is convincing evidence that strong connections can contribute to a long, healthy and happy life. Other studies show that individuals with strong social connections are 50% less likely to die prematurely. Being in a relationship adds 3 years on average to life expectancy.

They help us experience less stress. Social connections help us cope with stress. The kind of support and consideration a friend offers may serve as a safeguard, shielding us against the effects of stress. They help us stay healthier, not only in the long but also in the short run. According to a study by psychologist Sheldon Cohen, students who reported having strong connections were also more resilient to the flu virus.

Loneliness, on the other hand, is associated with depression and sickness. Lack of social connections can cause many problems related to physical, emotional and mental health. Isolation is fatal.

Indeed, all we need is love. When we are among friends, when we feel loved, a special hormone in our brain is released: Oxytocin. It is known as the "love hormone" or the "childbirth hormone" (since it is released during childbirth). Oxytocin contributes to good health: it is associated with lowering blood pressure and supressing stress hormones. It calms us down, generates a pleasant state of mind, renders a sense of trust and reduces depression.

The advantages are clear. Yet, not all are satisfied with the state of their social life and connections. The key is in prioritizing social connections, pulling away from destructive connections and investing in establishing new or nurturing existing ones. Beyond examining the social connections you have and the degree of support they afford you, the way to sustain connections and make them stronger is simply to invest in them: give more of yourself, make more opportunities for getting together, make the call, write a letter. The idea is to preserve and enhance those connections you have with the people who are dear to you and who hold you dear. Yet another option is to seek new social circles at work, at school and so forth.

As Ralph Waldo Emerson once said,

"The only way to have a friend is to be one. Make yourself necessary to somebody."

Would you like some Oxytocin to be released now? Oxytocin is released during an orgasm, though I am not sure how politically correct it is to send you off to make love at this moment. Nevertheless, Oxytocin is also released during a hug, a massage or while listening to cheerful music. Studies show that Oxytocin is also released when being out in nature listening to its sounds, such as bird song or the sound of the sea.

Which option do you choose?

Leisure/ Creativity/Personal Development

"Time is really the only capital that any human being has and the thing that he can least afford to waste or lose."

Thomas Edison

Leisure

It is tempting (almost impossible to resist) to join the endless race for happiness, money and career. Moreover, it is easy to sink into and get stuck in a daily rut, going from one chore to the next, forgetting that every day presents an opportunity to make progress on personal development, to experience, discover and do something new.

Leisure is time not dedicated to essential activities such as earning a living or social and familial obligations. Leisure is time that can be devoted to your hobbies — not done as an imperative but rather out of choice.

Leisure activities are paramount to our wellbeing. They bring about joy and generate a sense of balance, allow us to enjoy ourselves and learn at the same time — could there be a better combination? Leisure activities are an excellent opportunity for us to celebrate our successes and give ourselves simply time to have fun.

Dr Robert Stebbins, a world-renowned leading sociologist in the field of leisure studies, whose observations are based on decades of research, speaks of the Homo Otiosus (leisure man). He makes an interesting distinction between occasional leisure activities and "serious leisure" activities. According to him, combining occasional leisure and serious leisure enables us to live positive, rewarding, valuable lives.

Occasional leisure activities are short-term activities. They do not require skill, investment of resources or effort. We do them simply to take a break: read a newspaper, watch television, surf the Web, play computer games, go to a restaurant, do shopping, chat with friends or just take a rest.

Serious leisure activities, in contrast, are those we take seriously, where we are meticulous about learning and developing skills, with the highest degree of commitment and dedication (so much so that we sometimes become bona fide professional experts).

What are your leisure activities? What other activities would you supplement them with for a richer experience of leisure? What hobby stirs passion and challenge in you to the point that you would like to turn it into a serious field of interest, one in which you get better and gain expertise?

Dr Stebbins's research from the past 40 years has demonstrated that people who are involved in serious leisure activities are happier and more satisfied. Leisure activities offer an opportunity for self-fulfilment and personal development, a way to experience challenge, progress, satisfaction and happiness.

This might sound good on paper, but in real life it might not seem logical or probable to set time aside especially for leisure. The first step is to intentionally free up time for yourself. This could be 10 minutes before going to bed so that you could read a book or schedule half an hour for a piano lesson. Once you free up time on your schedule just for leisure, you will find ways to fill it up with the right activities. Alternately, once you find a serious hobby you are hooked on, you will use every bit of time to practice it.

Creativity

Creativity is a source of nourishment in our lives, through which we give vent to feelings and desires within ourselves whether conscious or subconscious.

What inspires you? How would you feel if you allowed yourself more space for self-expression? How could you add more room in your life for creativity?

There are countless ways to add that creative spark to almost anything you do: while cooking, playing with your children, in the way you dress, at work, in dance, photography, painting and so forth.

Allow creativity to be a part of your life. Let it find expression without judgement or any other objectives other than setting it free. Creativity brings about happiness, a sense of satisfaction and new discoveries.

Personal Development

Personal development is a process of growth and empowerment on the way to realizing your potential. It helps you live a happier, more complete life, explore your higher self, learn and develop.

It is a process that will allow you to connect to your core essence, to discover the true self that hides within you. Throughout the process you will discover characteristics, qualities and skills within yourself. Such process of growth grants you the opportunity to overcome obstacles, limiting beliefs, regressive attitudes and fears, so that you may open yourself up to countless opportunities.

Various agents may support your personal development: participating in various workshops, reading books about personal development, taking sessions with a personal coach, listening to a spiritual guide and so on. These agents can encourage you to see various events in our life in a different light, change your perspective, raise your self-awareness and serve as a vehicle for change.

Personal development happens when you are exposed to new ideas, when you learn to see the world and yourself in new ways without hanging on to the past. The process requires letting go of patterns and habits that hold you back.

Regard the past not as a prison but as a school. Take in its lessons and move forward. Remember, your future is richer and greater than your past. Invest time, effort and money in yourself. Consider yourself as a serious project. You are the hero/heroine of your life story. You hold the key to your own health, happiness and success.

NLP

NLP is the acronym for Neuro-Linguistic Programming. The prefix "neuro" refers to neural pathways and the nervous system — the means through which we experience our surroundings and receive its messages. The word "linguistic" refers to language — the means by which we process those messages we incorporated from our environment and translate them into voiceless self-talk (our internal dialogue with ourselves) or voiced, that is, spoken communication (our communication with our environment). The word "programming" refers to the formation of cognitive and behavioural patterns that rely on language and neural pathways.

NLP connects to your subconscious and assists you in controlling cognitive patterns, so you can be master of your mood and the power stored in your thoughts.

The method — developed in the United States by the mathematician Dr Richard Bandler (who also happens to be the one who trained me in NLP) and the linguist Dr John Grinder — has proved very useful.

The method includes various techniques that will help you change your cognitions and behaviour. NLP is the source and basis of life coaching. With the help of NLP sessions, you could free yourself of negative memories, behavioural patterns, or thoughts or feelings that hold you back, and replace them with new, positive, healthy patterns. Considering health and wellbeing, NLP is conducive to preserving good health over time as well as to disease prevention.

NLP can be beneficial to physical conditions such as allergies and food intolerance. It can complement conventional course of treatments and expedite recovery. It can support coping with chronic, incurable diseases by slowing down their progress and learning how to come to terms with them. It can also assist you with weight loss. It can promote coping with fear or stress.

NLP can help you get unstuck in life in situations that concern your job or your relationship. It can spur a genuine breakthrough in self-fulfilment and personal growth.

5 Keys to Happiness

Our physical and emotional health is important to us. When we are happy we take better care of ourselves and those around us, and we make better choices. Happiness fills us with energy and efficiency — we simply enjoy life better.

Harvard psychologist Shawn Achor, who advocates for positive psychology, tells us on his TED talk about the 5 keys to happiness. I will gladly share them with you here. Perhaps you will find one of them (or more) useful and take upon yourself the 21-day challenge. Following these guidelines for 21 days in a row will lead to a profound change to your thought patterns as well as generate positive thinking, will train your brain to be more positive, will raise your general level of positivity, creativity, energy and efficiency.

There is general understanding of happiness as external when it is pushed behind success, in fact, when it is made to depend on success. Achor suggests turning this formula upside down, training the brain to be happy regardless of external factors. He claims exercising this formula repeatedly helps to release the hormone Dopamine in our brain. This neurological process works on two different levels: it makes us happier and it turns on our learning capabilities and helps us be more receptive, efficient, open and motivated in absorbing information.

Here is his formula for positivity and happiness in 21 days:

1. 3 Gratitudes — the practice of expressing gratitude for three new things every day. It trains our brain to first seek the positive, not the negative.

2. Journaling — the practice of writing in a personal diary about one positive experience we have had in the past 24 hours. It allows us to relive it.

3. Exercise — teaches our brain that our behaviour is important. It matters.

4. Meditation — helps us cope with multi-tasking culture (the collective societal ADHD we have been creating). It helps us focus and soothes our mind.

5. Random acts of kindness — acts of generosity and kindness towards someone in our social network (a family member, a colleague, a friend).

If you decide to take on the 21-day challenge, I would love to hear of your experience — how it has affected your positivity and success in life. Please write to me at nellylewiscentre@gmail.com.

How Can Life-style Coaching Help?

If your health is important to you, and you feel you need help improving your health, there are probably reasons why this book has made its way to you. I truly hope you found in it vital information and inspiration to live a better life.

In our world, loaded with distractions, processed food, long sessions in front of the computer and long commutes, it is not always easy to establish a healthy lifestyle in every respect. Even when you have a clear idea of your weak points and goals — what lifestyle and health choices you wish for yourself — the path to making them come true can be long and difficult. Even when you know what you would like to do, falling back on old habits is easy, though change may be relatively easy to accomplish. Sometimes it turns out it is easier not to do.

Not every individual is well suited for coaching. First, you need to want it — set your heart on change, improvement, learning and growth, assuming active responsibility for your lifestyle. The process of coaching begins from your determined resolution to invest yourself in your own progress. Coaching can help you achieve your goals more easily, and much faster, compared to doing it on your own without professional support.

Coaching, as a profession, was born out of the need to create an alternative for or support the conventional health system, which usually puts an emphasis on symptoms rather than the human being as a whole. Studies demonstrate that most diseases that affect life quality and health are the result unhealthy choices (smoking, unhealthy nutrition, stress and so on). The conventional health system does not address the healthy individual who makes unhealthy daily choices that eventually lead to sickness. This is a crucial point. From this standpoint, coaching may be regarded as preventative healthcare, a type of proactive health insurance.

When I speak of a healthy lifestyle, I do not refer to a rigid series of rules but to a way of life in which you feel yourself to be strong and in control of your health choices — the master of your body and soul. The steps you take along the way are small, consistent steps. As your coach, I hold you accountable to your actions. In fact, the most important role of coaching is to make sure you follow up on your goals within the timeframe you set for yourself — no excuses. Once you zero in on your goals, once you know which steps you would like to take to accomplish them, I, as your coach, do the outmost to assist you in fulfilling them.

The coach-coachee relationship is a special one. It involves no judgement, only immense support. Your coach believes in you and sees windows of opportunities and possibilities within your reach, perhaps more than you can. Such faith gives wing to your efforts and success. The key is in small steps that generate a natural process that takes hold over time.

Sessions takes place at the clinic, through Skype or over the phone. The process is focused and tailored to the coachee. It is designed to fit your circumstances, your goals and the choices you make for yourself.

The coaching experience is truly transformative. It does wonders in fulfilling a healthy lifestyle. Just as every key factor on the health chart is related to the other, so are the various factors in a coachee's life: work, self-fulfilment, family life and so forth. The combination of personal coaching, life-style coaching and NLP (as well as the vast information available on health) ensures an enriching, conducive and healing experience.

Whether you feel your health condition would benefit from coaching or you wish to celebrate life by boosting your healthy lifestyle, I would gladly be there for you.

It will be a great privilege to be your companion on your journey to attain better health.

I invite you to visit my website www.nellylewis.com and get in touch.

"She turned her can'ts into cans and her dreams into plans."

Kobi Yamada, "She"